# Obsessive Compulsive Disorder Explained

OCD Facts, Diagnosis, Symptoms, Treatment, Causes, Effects, Alternative Medicines, Therapeutic Methods, History, Home Remedies, and More!

By  Frederick Earlstein

# Foreword

Obsessive - Compulsive Behavior is one among the 20 causes of disability worldwide, according to the World Health Organization's recent mental health reports. It was reported that OCD is the fourth most typically diagnosed mental illness trailing major depression, phobias, drug and alcohol abuse.

OCD can prevent a person from functioning normally in the world, so it is very important recognize not only the symptoms but also when to get help and see a specialist. OCD can rob someone of the quality of life many of us take for granted. There are available tests to determine if a person has OCD, there are also available medications, and therapies which a person or a family member can look into to get help from experts, and this book can help you to not just understand the disorder but also help you figure out how you can alleviate it and prevent symptoms from happening as much as possible.

# Table of Contents

# Introduction

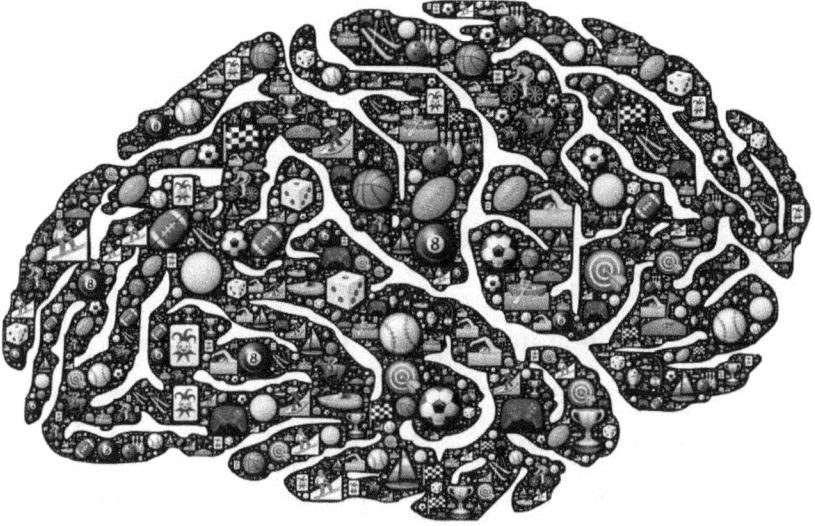

A condition that has been often times ridiculed and set to laughter in movies and misunderstood by people in general, OCD has been belittled and pooh-poohed by many. OCD needs to be understood properly in order for a sufferer of the disorder to know where their behavior is coming from and identify it for what it is so as to get the proper help they may need.

Research has shown that the brain disorder, OCD is the result of incorrect process of information in the brain. OCD patients say that it's their behavioral condition could be likened to a broken record being stuck on a specific thought. Although once believed to have no treatment, the advances in technology have greatly increased.

Not to be taken lightly, OCD is a very real, very limiting condition that many people suffer from which, when at its most severe, interrupts and intrudes with the quality of lives of those suffering from the it. Even the mildest conditions affect people with OCD. A lot of these obsessive and or compulsive behaviors can get in the way of the daily routine of a patient suffering from the disorder.

Obsessive Compulsive Disorder (OCD) is a neurological condition that compels a patient, who suffers from it, to do things which would seem strange, unusual and unnecessary to an onlooker. The person suffering from it may or may not be aware of the fact that these are unnecessary movements, actions or tasks but are nonetheless compelled to carry them out completing repetitive actions to satisfy their sense of balance even for just a little while.

We shall also be looking into the obsessive behaviors a person could suffer in silence to have you, our reader know more about the challenges an OCD patient goes through. We shall learn of medication and treatments which are available to the patient. We also want to be able to point you toward the right direction in order to get help and treatment for the disorder.

Let us delve in and look into the different degrees and severity of the condition and discover what the signs are in order for you to be aware of clues present and displayed by an individual with OCD. We aim to help you find out about all the symptoms so as you may be able to identify the red flags. This book is not only aimed to help a sufferer from the disorder to recognize signs and symptoms, it is also geared to enlighten friends and family members of sufferers of OCD.

# Chapter One: What is OCD?

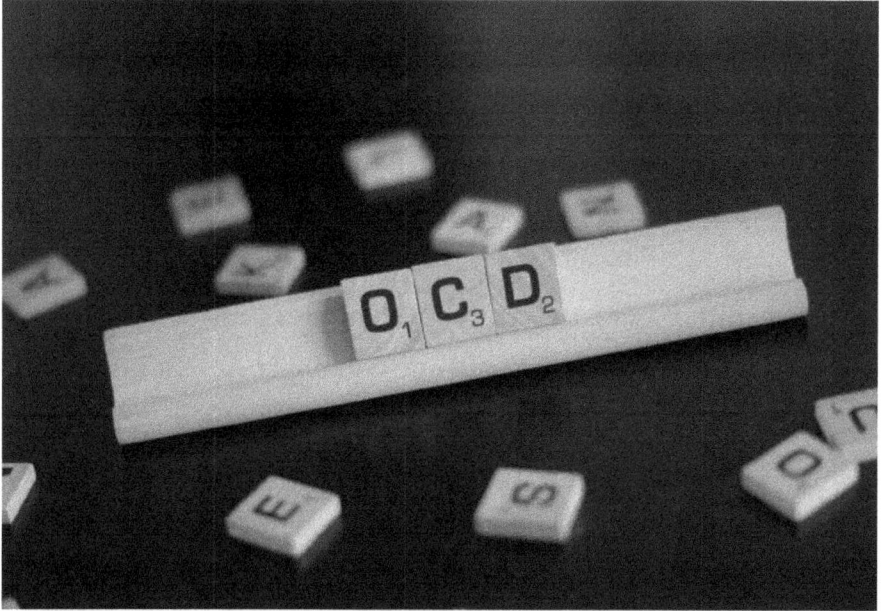

Obsessive-Compulsive Disorder (OCD) is a chronic condition which compels an individual suffering from it to do things repeatedly which is classified as compulsions while another person with OCD could have obsessive disturbing thoughts that run through their minds. It is a long-lasting disorder that is common in people and usually detected in persons at a young age. This chapter will delve deeper on what this disorder is all about.

*Facts about OCD*

Some experts say that OCD could be genetic and inherited; others believe that it is a trauma based disorder which gets triggered off by a highly stressful or traumatic experience. And there are those who say that both are true.

Either way, the truth of the matter is these obsessive thoughts and or compulsive behaviors have a great likelihood of interrupting the lives of patients who have been diagnosed with it and most especially those who have been left unchecked and undiagnosed. A patient may display symptoms of both obsessive and compulsive behaviors or they may display symptoms of only one or the other.

An individual with OCD may show more telling signs when they obsess about cleanliness and hygiene. What, to others, are natural and normal things required of them to do to go about their day, an OCD patient may find repulsive and repugnant. For some patients the mere thought of opening a door appalls them to their core that they would wait until someone else came along to do it. The fear of catching or get infected by a virus to them is a deep seated fear which they cannot help and some would try to find ways to cope with their OCD in their own ways - ways that are somehow strange to those around them.

Patients of OCD have been known to wash their hands repeatedly or compulsively use hand sanitizers which they carry around with them at all times, everywhere. Others have been observed to wear gloves and a face mask for fear of getting infected with germs, perhaps by people they may come in close contact or from the environment in which they need to move about. They are afraid to touch things or people with their bare hands and all of that can become quite overwhelming for them as it becomes frustrating for those around them.

Some need perfect symmetry in everything around them that they go around fixing things that they feel are off kilter, out of place or balance, tilted or crooked. There are patients who would line up their clothes in their dressers according the shades and hues of the textile. In others, the disorder is exhibited in the patient as unwanted thoughts, disturbing yet fleeting images of doing or causing harm on themselves or someone else. Others would feel compelled to count repeatedly, then there are those who would check, recheck and go back to check that they have locked all their windows and doors.

Those with ritualistic behaviors find no pleasure in the actions they carry out but in their minds these are necessary things to do in order to get their world in order. They find fleeting relief in the comforting, assuring, ritualistic actions they carry out. People who have a hard time controlling their train of thought is asymptomatic of the behavioral disorder.

There are those who display the disorder as motor tics through vocal tics like throat clearing, snort, grunts, sniffing, coughing. These are sudden, jerky movements, eye blinking or fast eye movements, they repeatedly shrug their shoulders, grimace, shake or nod their heads.

People with OCD, whether they know it or not, may attempt "to cure" themselves by not getting into situations which they recognize as triggers. Others use drugs to calm themselves and then there are those who resort to the bottle. Almost all adults with OCD recognize the fact that the things they do don't make sense. In children it would usually be the parents or the child's teachers, who would recognize the manifestation of symptoms of disorder in the child.

OCD can prevent a person from functioning normally in the world, so it is very important recognize not only the symptoms but also when to get help and see a specialist. OCD can rob someone of the quality of life many of us take for granted. There are available tests to determine if a person has OCD. There is available medication, and therapy which a person or a family member can look into to get help from experts.

## How to tell if it is OCD?

We are all individuals with varied ways of dealing with everyday routine. There are many and varied reasons for an individual with OCD to get set off. It could be a big role change, like a promotion or having a baby. There is also a possibility of a serotonin imbalance in an individual which could be the culprit of OCD.

The meticulous personality of person who likes things in a certain order could seem like a good thing at first but could easily lead to OCD if not taken in to check. The things a person with OCD is compelled may seem mad to others and other people in the family may start to have upset days when they are directly involved with the OCD.

There are other conditions which mimic the symptoms of OCD such as the following:

- Tourette syndrome is where the patient has an uncontrollable urge to shout out expletives or make seemingly rude noises in the middle of a conversation or just out of the blue.

- When a person is distressed about they look or a condition called body dysmorphic disorder a person becomes convinced of something off in their looks and obsess about their appearance, always finding some sort of fault with the way they look.

- A compulsion to pull out one's hair or eyebrows is a condition Trichotillomania is another condition which mimics the symptoms of OCD.

- Hypochondria is when a patient is in constant fear about being infected by a disease or virus stemming from an experience perhaps they may have experienced in their lifetime.

- A form of autism called Asperger's syndrome is another condition whose symptoms of needing to do the same things over and over again becomes a compulsion.

- Depression and anxiety and a handful of other mental related health issues can also be part of, accompanied by, or the start of OCD.

## OCD in Women, Men and Children

Women, men and children all over the world are affected by obsessive compulsive disorder and may not know it. Many of them left unchecked due to poor health care or unrecognized symptoms. Most people affected in developed countries are diagnosed in their teens. These cases are usually suspected by and identified by constant guardians, like parents and teachers. 2 - 3% of adults and children will be diagnosed with OCD. More adult women are affected by OCD than men, but it was noted that childhood OCD is more prevalent in boys than it is in girls.

Obsessive thoughts could be based on the strong beliefs, standards and or morality of a person with OCD of which they hold themselves up to. It is specific to each individual but this has a recurring pattern of violence, destruction or injury, and even killing. These dark thoughts spin into guilty feelings and anxiety for the impending present and the turnout of events in the near future.

Young people, for fear of being excluded and shunned by their peers struggle to find ways to control and manage their behavioral ticks and intrusive mind images. This can be detrimental to the young person's wellbeing as they would usually withdraw into themselves afraid of being found out and labeled, making it harder to identify the symptoms and getting help for the individual. It is very important to be able to get help for a young adult as such so they are able to relieve themselves of the burden of feeling different and alone.

There is a diagnostic criteria doctor and experts use these days to diagnose OCD. Not guaranteeing cure, there are treatments which in fact heave helped many OCD sufferers allowing them to live a good quality of life. There is available medication to help severe and moderate OCD as well as therapy to allow the individual to work through their issues with an expert.

CBT is a psychotherapeutic method which has been proven to control and manage OCD. Another form of therapy is ERP or Exposure and Response Prevention, classified as a CBT therapy, involves the OCD patient to be exposed to the obsessed upon feared object or situation

## Forms of Severe and Mild OCD

It is safe to say that there are mild and severe cases of OCD afflicting a multitude of people. Some of them have the milder effect of the disorder but can equally be a bother to them. Those who understand and recognize the disorder are usually those who have reached out and gotten help and have been able to manage their days with prescribed medication, therapy or the combination of both. And then there are those on the fringes of society who have no idea what OCD is who live lives of accepted ridicule. Going about and managing their days as best they can. The onset of OCD can happen early in a young person's life from 7 to 12 years old and then there are times when the behavioral disorder is displayed by a young teenager.

Overall, most men and women are generally aware of when their condition began or at what age they started showing symptoms. Many recognize their actions and thoughts but are not able to control themselves. Those with motor tics often have a difficult time finishing a sentence until they have, say, jerked their shoulders or head a specific number of times. Others are snorters, who would either snort out their breath a certain number of times before allowing themselves to calm for a moment and breathe normally. Others are grunters, needing to make a throaty sound before spitting out the rest of their sentence vocally.

The compulsion may change over the course of time depending on the severity of the case. There are those who are able to handle their condition and manage it with help and strong will. It could ease up over time or go a totally different direction - whether one compulsion is replaced by another or the condition worsens and totally disrupts the way of living of the individual as well as affecting lives of those around them.

One could identify symptoms in their children if a child insists on having their toys, clothes, shoes, or books arranged in a particularly specific manner and has a hard time accepting any proposed or carried out changes in said perfect arrangement.

At its most severe, OCD can be quite debilitating in a manner that the person suffering from the disorder is not able to carry out tasks routine, standard and considered to be regular to most people. At its worst people with severe

OCD can imagine imagines grim, dark and/or violent. They could imagine harming others in various ways and could also imagine hurting themselves.

Depending on the gravity of the illness in some people, patients may have a great fear of being contaminated by an unseen virus that could be carried and passed on by other people to them. In these severe cases, patients have been known to wash themselves immediately after an accidental or intended contact with another person or object. At times scrubbing their flesh raw until it bleeds, others with milder forms of contamination fear would constantly wash their hands or simply refuse to touch anything that other people have handled. It really does depend on the level of severity giving credence to the fact that there are milder and graver forms of OCD in twin observations.

The root of the obsession would seem very odd to a person who does not know the patient or who does not recognize the cause of the seeming misbehavior or quest for perfection. There are many facets and degrees to the behavioral disorder that it is important to know when to get help. And to know when to do that means to be able to recognize the symptoms. You have picked up this book to enlighten yourself more on the subject and our aim to shed light and reveal more of this common behavioral disorder.

# Chapter Two: Types of OCD

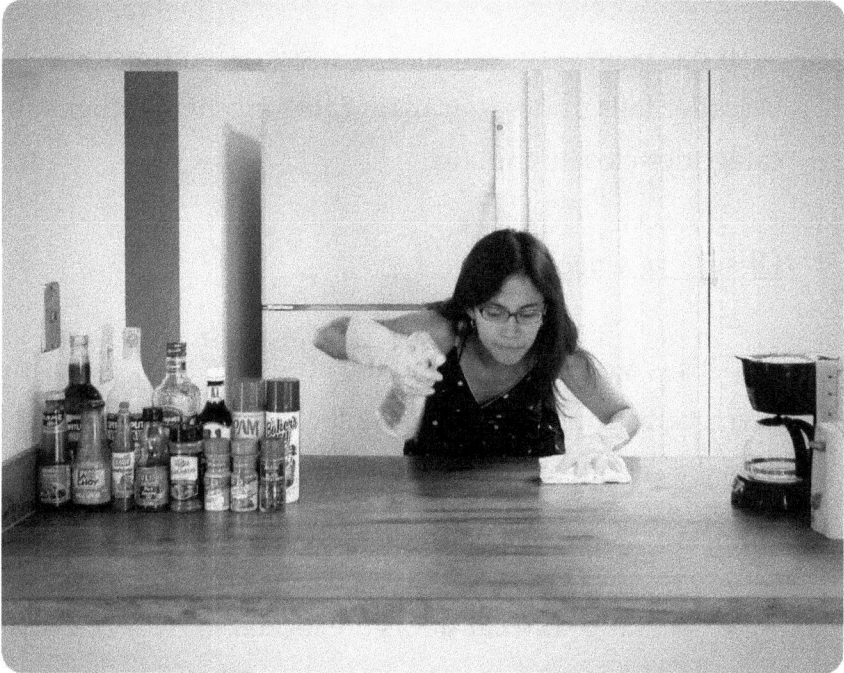

OCD has many facets to it and the symptoms and behaviors acted out are different for each individual who bears the illness. The fact that we now live in world where everything seems to be going too fast makes it even more difficult for the person with OCD to cope with the every demand of everyday and deal with their ailment. Should you suspect that you or a member of your family be suffering from OCD, it is important that it is discussed with a specialist, therapist or your family physician.

## Sub – Categories of OCD

It has been surmised that Obsessive Compulsive Disorder falls under four main categories with other sub-categories closely trailing.

### Obsessive Checking

This is a compulsion and the obsessive fear of causing harm, catastrophe or damage. One form is memory checking to make certain an uninvited thought is merely that and nothing more. Some of the more typical checking rituals are:

- Making sure car doors are locked for fear of causing falling accidents.

- Checking doors and windows are locked to prevent possible break - ins.

- Double checking appliances are off for fear of causing burning or injury.

- Wallets and purses are constantly checked to be there and not missing for fear of losing something important

- Calling people to check up on them and their safety. It is one thing to check in and have the person know they are fine, quite another thing when the phone rings off the hook.

- Fear of doing or saying something which may offend or upset a loved one, a family member or friends.

- Fear of OCD being the precursor to Schizophrenia causing the individual to lose control over themselves or their urges.

## Fear of Germ or Mental Contamination

This is the compulsion of the patient to clean and wash themselves or things other people may have handled which may contaminate them causing sickness, disease and/or death of self or a loved one. Some people with OCD could potentially get sick physically because of this constant fear of being contaminated with germs. Take for example a person who won't do nature's business outside of their home. Holding in one's urge to urinate because of public toilets can be detrimental to their health and cause great anxiety for the person and those around them.

Other people are afraid to shake hands for fear of contracting the germs of another. Waiting in the office of a doctor can cause great anxiety to some OCD patients due to the idea that there may be one who has a communicable disease which can be contracted if airborne. Other people have a great repulsion about visiting hospitals for fear of being exposed to sickness. Touching banisters, staircases, hand railings, doorknobs and a toilet flush are other forms of fear of contamination.

Fear of contamination can be a real problem for the individual as in most these cases people with this OCD will act accordingly and avoid these situations making it hard for them to go out of the house, be around people or hold a job.

Mental contamination is an OCD symptom that is less obvious, share particular qualities with contact contamination but with its own distinct and set apart features. These are intrusive thoughts brought about by times when a person felt ill-treated, whether mentally or physically. It could stem from being criticized, mentally or verbally abused. This is when the person feels they have been treated unfairly, like something disposable, creating a feeling of being unclean internally.

Mental contamination is quite distinct because the source of this is human, not like fear of germ contamination where the contaminant is caused by touching objects handled by others.

## Hoarding

This is the inability to get rid of acquired possessions and the inability to control oneself from getting and keeping more things than they can afford, house or store. Hoarding becomes not only the problem of the OCD patient but ultimately becomes part of the everyday lives of their family and friends around them. It is not unusual for hoarders to become recluse if not given treatment or help. They understand that their actions are unreasonable and unnecessary but they are compelled to do so because of lack of treatment and discussion with a person who understands and is willing to help the patient get help.

## Rumination / Intrusive Imaginings

These are not merely thought of fleeting but more poignant, more thoughtful questions that are difficult to answer. Some of the things people ruminate about are questions like what happens after death? Is there good in everyone? Are some people innately evil? These become OCD symptoms because of the time spent pondering on these thoughts that have no defined answers.

In the spectrum of OCD Intrusive Imaginings are images of violence in person's mind's eye causing harm or danger to loved ones. These thoughts which come involuntarily are repetitive thoughts that cause great distress to the individual. It is however known factually that a person with OCD is the least likely to cause any violence to anyone they love or anyone else for that matter.

These four areas are most common sorts of OCD as well as some of the associated fears which come along with them. This is by no means the only behavioral and ritualistic actions as there are other sub-categories of the ailment.

# Chapter Three: Signs and Symptoms, Diagnosis and Treatments

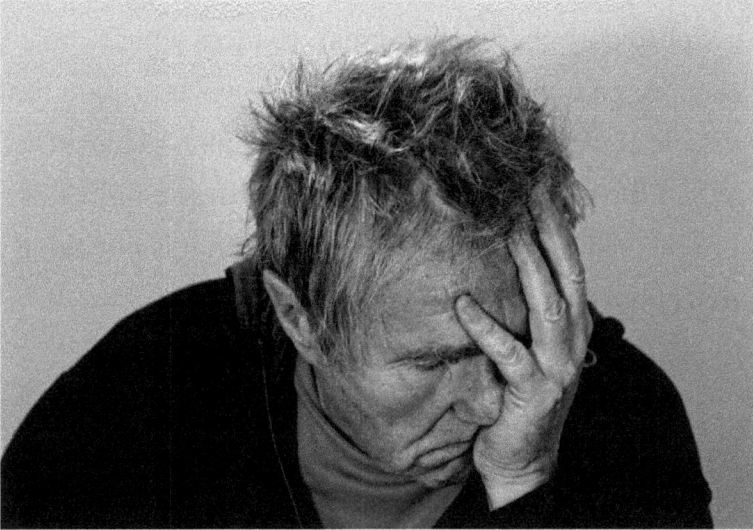

When a person's thought pattern is interrupted with unreasonable fears, disturbing images, thoughts or urges which cause the patient anxiety and or when the person in question is compelled to do things repetitively, these are signs and symptoms of the behavioral disorder. Typically considered a lifelong behavior disorder that can range from mild to severe, OCD can be manageable if detected and diagnosed early. It is true that a sufferer of the disorder can live a normal life mingled with society if given the help they need. In this chapter, you'll learn the symptoms, diagnosis and the treatments available to better manage the disorder.

## Signs and Symptoms

Compulsions are ritualistic actions a patient performs in order to curb these mental disturbances which make them seem to go unhinged to the trained eye. It is often times visible clues that would suggest a person to have OCD. When the OCD patient internalizes these patterns of unreasonable thoughts are times when it is not as easy to detect the cues.

Perhaps noticeable through actions unnecessary, to what we would consider as the usual method of order, some patients would exhibit excessive obsession in the "little" things. Take for example cleanliness. They may take time brushing one tooth at a time, paying close mind to the number of cleaning brush strokes, displaying worry about their dental hygiene. Others may display symptoms through cleaning sprees, making sure that each nook and cranny of a space is dusted, wiped down, cleaned and disinfected. Others may need things in a certain order or pattern before they are able to do anything else. Like let's say, a child who needs to do their homework would first need to have everything around her in order and in its proper place. This may give her the balance she needs to start focusing on the first needful task properly.

Not to say that if you are a ritualistic cleaner, you may have OCD. As human beings mature, we carry out actions to master these everyday routine skills to somehow take hold of the reins of our lives, that it becomes second nature. But it has been observed that a steady and strengthening rise of these compulsive or obsessive behaviors in a small number of young ones turn out to become rigid expectations.

Harder to identify are the mental rituals people deal with on a daily basis. Some of the more common in some patients are fleeting imaginings in their head that would set off anxiety in them, thoughts and mental images of killing, death, and mayhem - just general chaos and violence.

Anchored also in superstition, the patient may begin to chant a prayer or repeat phrases to "ward off that evil thought" and attempt to calm themselves down this way. Others are very visible and not only affect the person with the disorder but also the people around them.

Not unusual to a growing OCD patient or young adolescent is the shift of themes as they grow. Subjects relevant to their age range and belief systems, such as topics on religion, sex, sexuality, moral concerns incorporate and mingle. Therefore it is important for the patients to get the help they need because not only can the behavioral disorder become crippling, this can be quite disconcerting to an individual who is experiencing OCD but does not know it.

## What Triggers OCD?

To some the thought of touching something another person has touched utterly repulses them because of contamination fear. Others see disorder when things are not facing a certain manner or arranged according to their order bringing to mind Monica Geller and her obsession about having everything in its place to keep her world in order.

People with OCD may attempt to stop these obsessions but it just heightens their anxiety and distress driving them to carry out acts of compulsion to ease out their stress and smooth the kinks often centering on themes privy to them or to select people closest to them. One thing common amongst OCD patients is their fear of losing it and losing control of themselves, but this is so far from the truth. Historically, people with OCD are not capable of actually carrying out unimaginable violence.

There are a number of reasons and theories to the onset of OCD in individuals. There are those who say that it is a genetic disorder inherited from one generation to another. Then there are experts who say that the behavioral disorder is acquired after a sudden, often traumatic experience and is used by an individual as a way to cope with the anxiety driven situation and inadvertently cause episodes thereafter.

## Diagnosis

In order to rule out other underlying medical issues if any, your doctor may ask you to undergo a physical exam where your blood will be test. This is usually a CBC or a complete blood count. They may check out the function of your thyroid and screen you for drugs and alcohol. It is helpful to have a close relation like a family member or friend to whom you can confide but you have to know when you need to consult with experienced medical professionals. There is no reason to keep OCD a secret and bear with the burden of how taxing it can get. There are available methods to help a person with OCD live a good quality of life and function well in society. Expect a psychological evil and be ready to hash out your thoughts, emotions, feelings, as well as your behavioral patterns to a doctor.

## When to See a Doctor

There are mild forms of OCD that can be managed through specific methods aided or not by medication and allow an individual suffering from it live a close to normal life. Others are moderate forms to severe cases of OCD that make it difficult for the individual to function properly because of the consumption of time it takes them to ease and calm themselves, pretty much disabling themselves from performing everyday tasks.

If a person shows signs of worsening OC behavioral disorder, it is time to look for a specialist if you haven't got one already. Some mild cases seem to disappear in its own and the patient is able to manage their lives. Once your quality of life is affected, like not being able to show up for work on time because of the many rituals you need to perform before even starting your day, it is time to get help.

Not only can this be disabling to you but also the people around you. Some OCD patients especially those who are younger and have limited capacity for vocabulary and explaining the way they feel, are especially concerning because it causes anxiety to parents when there is in fact several ways of managing the disorder. Performance like the act of getting out of the house can become a chore in itself to a person with OCD, as they make sure that everything that needs to be switched off, or turned off. It's one thing when a person does this on a frazzling day just to make sure that everything is on the up and up. It is quite a different thing when the time consuming, repetitive actions get in the way of the person's life.

It seems that there is a stronger likelihood for children of adults with OCD to have them as well. Studies and observations have shown that OCD can in fact be inherited from either parent who has OCD. It has also been noted that symptoms of OCD behavior can display itself soon after a traumatic experience which triggers off uninvited imaginings and worrying distress to the individual.

The simple actions and routine of life becomes taxing and demanding, making it difficult for the patient to live life to its fullest.

## *Treatments*

There is definitely help out there for those who are seeking confirmation of condition and who want to be able to manage the disorder. Being one of the more common behavioral disorders found in about 1 of 50 people, you can be sure that you are not alone.

Having been able to identify a chemical imbalance of serotonin has allowed medical experts come up with medication that can help balance out the lack of this chemical in an OCD patient. There are also a number of psychiatric therapy methods aimed at empowering an individual with OCD overcome their fear of whatever they are compelled or obsessed about.

### **Psychotherapy**

Knowing what you are going through and that you are not alone is an empowering feeling of being to take some control over the disorder. It may make you feel embarrassed at first or defensive about your condition but it is important to get the help you need and map out a treatment plan. Consider joining a support group who face the same challenges, it is important for you to know that the struggle is real and you don't have to go at it on your own. Some conditions are more severe than others and hence it is advisable to know where to get long-term group care in order to cope better.

Stay goal oriented and never lose sight of your recovery goals. Keep in mind that overcoming OCD is a goal to be made one day at a time. It is an ongoing process for some of the more moderate to severe cases.

## Psychosurgery

There are severe cases when patients do not respond to behavioral therapy or medications to alleviate OCD symptoms and psychosurgery are used. There are four kinds of brain surgery that have been proven effective in the treatment of OCD according to the International OCD Foundation.

Anterior cingulotomy involves drilling a hole into the skull then burning an area of the brain known as the anterior cingulate cortex using a heated probe. This is the first form of psychosurgery which has given and shown positive benefits to 50% of OCD patients who initially displayed resistance to medical and therapy treatments.

Anterior capsulotomy another form of psychosurgery procedure similar to the first one mentioned above but another part of the brain is operated on called the anterior limb of the internal capsule. It has been documented that this surgery of burning a part of the brain with a hot probe has given 50 to 60 percent relief to patients who display resistance to the usual conventional treatments of OCD.

The gamma knife is the third sort of psychosurgery to treat OCD and does not require cracking open a patient's skull. Instead, the skull of the OCD patient is penetrated by gamma rays in high, multiple doses. A single dose of gamma ray will not make a dent of difference in harming brain matter. However this changes drastically when an intersection of multiple sources of gamma ray converge. When this happens, this creates energy that is enough to kill a target area of the brain. This procedure using gamma knife

rays has given relief to about 60 percent of OCD patients
who have shown resistance to treatments.

And lastly, available as well and something to discuss
with your doctor is the deep brain stimulation (DBS). This is
a procedure which requires operating and opening the
patient's skull but does not entail the destruction of brain
tissue. The procedure is instead done by using electrodes
which are strategically placed at specific points inside of the
brain and are in turn hooked up to a pulse generator. The
implantable neurostimulator is battery-powered generator,
which transmits pulses to the brain.

The implantable neurostimulator works a lot like a
pacemaker. There have only been a handful of studies on
deep brain stimulation but the response to the procedure has
been good, showing a same response rate to the other
surgeries available.

**Where to Find Treatment**

Your family physician is the first person outside of your
family who you want to talk to if you suspects OCD and
because it is a particular disorder needing specialized care.

Your doctor will be able to recommend specialists in the area with whom you could set an appointment. Since OCD symptoms have similarities with other neurological diseases like anxiety and depression and because the can be present alongside it, it will be important to discuss other existing mental health issues with a specialist.

## OCD Medications: Over-the-Counter and Prescription

Prescribed medication could potentially reduce symptoms of OCD from around 40 to 60 percent in most patients; this is according to the International OCD Foundation.

Most of the prescription drugs used in treating OCD is antidepressants, because often times, depression stems from the effects of OCD. One medication is enough to treat both disorders of OCD and depression; however, not all antidepressants work for OCD symptoms. Presently, there are several antidepressants which are known to work toward treating OCD and these drugs are Paroxetine (Paxil), Fluoxetine (Prozac), Escitalopram (Lexapro), Venlafaxine

(Effexor), Sertraline (Zoloft), Fluvoxamine (Luvox), Citalopram (Celexa), Clomipramine (Anafranil).

Already studied and tested on OCD patients, these antidepressants have been proven to work well in treating OCD. There have been case reports in the hundreds citing other prescription drugs which help treatment-resistant OCD patients but they need to be given in really high doses to show positive results toward treatment.

Never take antidepressants during stressful situations. This is a typical mistake of most patients who live with OCD. Doing so will not give you an instant gratification of solution to the immediate situation at hand. Instead an OCD patient needs to remember that antidepressants should be taken in prescribed doses consistently and should not be take outside of schedule. These are not to be taken like an anxiety medication.

Some patients could feel the immediate effects of antidepressants in a mere few days after taking these prescribed drugs. However, the result of the drugs in other patients can take up to as long as 10 to 2 weeks to display positive results.

For some people, they are able to cease taking the
antidepressants after a 12 month period. Then there are
those, approximately 50 percent of OCD patients, who must
maintain a certain dosage amount for an unspecified
number of years. Some will have to expect to take these
prescribed medications during their entire lives.

Medically Assisted OCD Therapy is available these days
to candidates who may want to sign up for them. Some of
the most commonly prescribed medications given to aid the
treatment of OCD in a patient are antidepressants clinically
known as selective serotonin reuptake inhibitors (SSRIs).
Should an OCD patient fail to respond to any of the SSRI
listed about, physicians turn to clomipramine. This is an
older tricyclic antidepressant which was the first prescribed
medication used for OCD treatment in the past.

It has greater efficacy than the rest of the aforementioned
medications we listed earlier but has side effects that can
become unpleasant to the patient. Sometimes and SSRI and
both used side by side as a combination drug to treat OCD.
Some of the side effects that follow clomipramine include a
drop in blood pressure when getting up from a lying or

seated posture, sleepiness, difficulty in releasing pee, cotton-mouth.

Atypical antipsychotics which have proven to be good for OCD in low doses are prescribed drugs like, Olanzapine, Ziprasidone, Risperidone and Quetiapine. Sometimes, there are cases where benzodiazepines can give relief to anxiety, but they are usually only used side by side with treatments that are reliable. Cognitive therapy is still the form of treatment best preferred by physicians; however a lot of patients gain positively from a combination of medication and therapy.

## Treatment Programs

There are other intensive treatment programs for those suffering with severe OCD available and which should be discussed. While some programs only last a weekend there are others which require the patient to a three-month stay at a treatment center. Individuals and OCD patients will undergo intensive individual, group and family cognitive therapy each day at these facilities. For those under the program a specifically devised medication regimen is also employed.

Presently there are other therapeutic methods, including studies involving the manipulation of neurotransmitters are in development and underway. Therefore there is absolutely no reason for anyone with OCD to continue to suffer or be immobilized by the disorder.

The use of electroconvulsive therapy (ECT), a procedure wherein the psychiatrist delivers tiny electric shocks to the patient's brain is in discussion at the National Alliance on Mental Illness (NAMI). The delivery of shock sets off a controlled seizure thereby activating neurons which helps bringing about changes in the patient's brain levels of neurochemicals making this a very effective method to manage and control OCD.

There is another process called Transcranial Magnetic Stimulation which uses magnetic fields. What is does is it stimulates the patient's brain nerve cells helping to decrease the intensity and severity of some of the symptoms of depression. It is the last resort most doctors employ when all other procedures do not seem to work.

## OCD Treatment Centers - Residential and Inpatient

In some cases, for patients who show very low or no
response to other therapies, residential and inpatient
treatment centers for OCD patients are available. These
treatment centers give residential and medical care, whilst
there are other treatment centers which also conduct
research on OCD therapies and treatments. Expect these
resident and inpatient centers to give structured, in-depth
therapy alongside psychopharmacological methods. Ask
about the varied methods employed by these individual
treatment centers and discuss these with your doctor. You
may also call any of the licensed treatment centers near your
area to know more about their methods

## Residential OCD Treatments - How Do You Benefit?

The good thing about residential OCD treatments is that
they are not just limited to intensive outpatient and inpatient
treatments because many of these residential treatment
facilities are in fact given value due to their research
programs. Aside from the important research geared toward
the treatment and therapy for OCD, these centres facilitate
and provide each patient with tailored programs fit for each

patient. Some of these OCD treatment centers offer intensive therapy alongside traditional care as well as diagnostics and treatments for comorbid conditions.

## OCD Disorder Luxury Facilities

Luxurious OCD treatment facilities have many luxury amenities much like forward-thinking rehabs. There are expert on hand staff members present along with gourmet chefs. It is located on pristine grounds and has some of the more exotic activities for the patients. Some are likened to spas and resorts, whilst some merge Eastern spiritual practices, like meditation activities and yoga sessions alongside with traditional therapy.

### Executive OCD Disorder Programs

There are also executive OCD programs which offer a great variety of top-notch amenities just like luxury facilities offering OCD treatments. These are geared more toward the treatment of corporate managers and business professionals who are not able to show up and stay for the residential program treatments and who require being able to go about business as usual alongside undergoing treatment.

## Treatment Programs for Outpatient OCD Rehab

Treatment programs for outpatient OCD rehabs provide some pretty intensive outpatient treatment supplied by staff members dedicated to helping the sufferers of OCD. They help patients and family with OCD and aim toward better management of the disorder, not only relevant for patients but also very useful and relevant to family members of the patient. A lot of these facilities do research and studies into OCD and employ research-based treatment options.

## Finding the Best OCD Treatment Facility

Aside from checking with your local mental health facilities on getting optimal OCD treatment, you can discuss your options about treatments and work hand in hand with your psychiatrist. Your doctor might be able to help you find the best OCD facilities in your area or in other locales that you can easily visit.

## What to Talk About With Your Doctor?

The aim essentially is to discuss the best medication for each individual. There is no one size-fits-all prescription. Some patients would do well without medication but will undergo therapy. Others are more receptive to doses of medication. Then there are those who respond better to both.

Ideally the aim is to identify medication which targets the need of each individual at the lowest possible dosage. There will be a big likelihood of trying out several drugs before you find the proper kind that will help manage the condition. This is why it is very important to be under the supervision of a doctor. It is possible for a doctor to prescribe more than one drug to manage the OCD symptoms better and it may take more than a couple of months to see positive results.

Another reason why it is important to be under the care and supervision of a doctor when undergoing medication is because of the side effects that may come along with the drugs. Drugs interacting with each other are not unusual since we are all made up differently. Some of these drugs will be anti-depressants and there is a suicide risk in young people and adults who are on it especially for the first few weeks after taking them. Suicidal thoughts are said to also happen when the dosage is changed. The risk doubles exponentially when the medication is suddenly ceased.

Discontinuation syndrome is a physical dependence on the prescribed medication aimed at OCD. This is very different from addiction but has withdrawal-like appearances. Even if you are feeling well, it is not advisable and risky to cease taking medication without discussing it first with your physician. You will need the supervision of your doctor so that they can help you lower and decrease your dosage gradually over time.

Mixing prescribed medications with herbal supplements and other mind impairing substances such as alcohol or street drugs is very dangerous. It is certainly not wise to do this but it is still something you want to be honest about with your doctor. There are patients who do not respond to medication and or psychotherapy and research continues toward deep brain stimulation to treat OCD. Those who do not respond to the usual approach of treatment could discuss DBS as an option with their doctor.

# Chapter Four: Lifestyle and Home Remedies for OCD

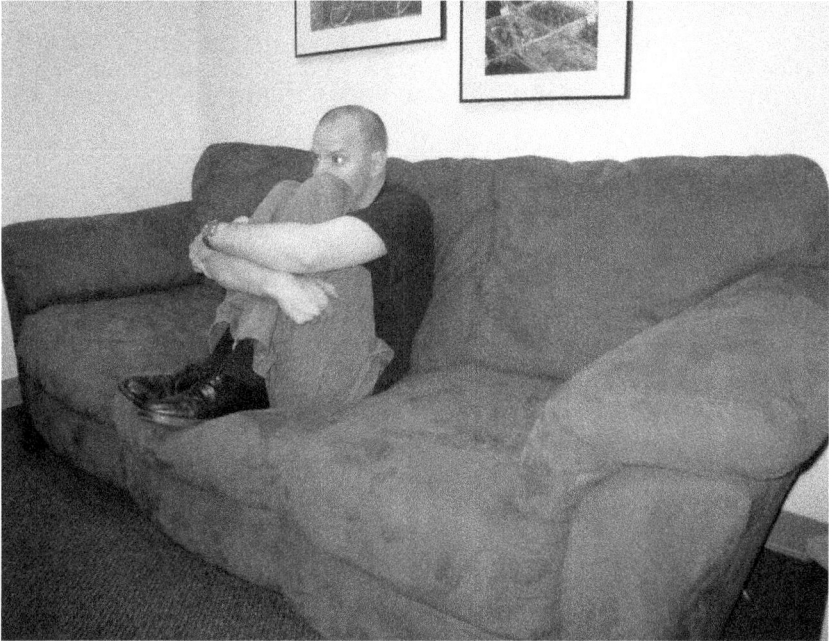

Keep your eye on the prize and set realistic goals for yourself. Look for healthy ways to occupy your time. Make it a point to exercise regularly. Eat healthy and make good dietary choices try to stick to a decent hour of sleep and get a full night's rest. When we begin to understand a disability we may possess it is important to become proactive and live consciously healthy lifestyles. This chapter will give some recommended foods that can help you alleviate the symptoms and make you live a healthier life.

## Tips for a Better Lifestyle

We adjust our lifestyles to aid health on when we are physically ill, so it makes no sense to not do the same when we face mental health challenges. When we are physically ill we are strongly advised by our doctors to get rid of one vice or another, eat better, sleep better, etc. So it is for OCD. The stigma attached to a person facing mental issues should be a thing of the past. Sadly, many are still in the dark about it. Go the whole nine yards and be your own cheerleader. Rally all the way and do not eliminate the fact that a good diet also equates to sound mental wellness.

Make an effort to live a regular lifestyle. Pay close mind that you keep schedules, show up for work, attend school and most importantly therapy sessions and doctor's appointments. Keep yourself surrounded with a solid support group. Be around supportive, well-versed in the disorder family and friends. Be able to recognize and identify signs of withdrawal whether mentally or physically. Your medication, if any, may be the culprit for depression or suicidal thoughts.

There are many community activities you can join that you can attend, sometimes for free other times at price less than private classes. Make sure to live in the moment and understand that you are able and can overcome whatever tick, image, or thought begin to try to overpower you. There are yoga, meditation, and group sessions to help you manage anxiety. Take advantage of these.

## Home Remedies to Treat OCD

Obsessive compulsive disorder has proven to be an illness that has affected many lives. And it spares no one, whether rich, poor, old and young. It is defined just as it is named and is characterized by symptoms of ritualistic, repetitive actions like knob turning, frequent hand washing, switching lights off and on and can sometimes be accompanied by nervous tics such as shoulder rotations, arm extensions, facial expressions and a host of other habits and tics. It is followed by anxious thoughts and feelings of panic which compel the sufferer to perform anxious ritualistic actions, which takes a lot of time from the person and sometimes the people around them, in order
to feel temporary relief or a sense of balance.

With the time spent on these response actions, the person's quality of life suffers because of the disorder. Most if not all patients suffering from OCD realizes that their actions are irrational but they can't help the strong need to do these. Having no clear known cause for the disorder, OCD is usually treated by means of medication and CBT. Since it happens over a vast spectrum severity, treatments can be different for each individual.

We aim to look for other ways and avenue a person could take in battling, managing and controlling the disorder hence we shall be looking into other ways that could help an individual help themselves with some remedies that can be readily available to them outside of the ususal drugs prescribed for OCD. And because of the variables of OCD, many people suffering from the disorder has looked at home remedies and natural ways to get rid of the symptoms of OCD in order to help them improve their way of living. We will be looking at some of the alternative, home remedies for OCD this time.

**Limiting Alcohol and Caffeine Intake**

Cut back on stress-inducing substances like alcohol and caffeine. Some people have mistakenly turned to alcohol and caffeine to try to bear down on the symptoms of OCD.

The issue with these chemical inducing substances is that once the rush of caffeine or alcohol wears out the patient is left with either a hangover or become jittery because of the amount of caffeine in their system leaving the individual in a state of lackluster. This could cause greater anxiety which sets off the OCD symptoms in high gear making it difficult for the patient to operate and go about their day even further.

## Schedule and Stick to Meal Times

People's bodies react negatively when under stress, deficient of nutrients or when hungry, which can result to an anxious mindset and increased stress levels. Make sure that you eat healthy and on time each day to prevent the onset of anxiety and stress. Low blood sugar causes body stress, aiding OCD symptoms along. Binge eating as well as eating your food in a hurry only makes matters worse and is not recommended. Be sure that you eat three square meals a day, taking care to chew on your food thoughtfully and carefully.

## Marijuana

More and more studies are coming out on the benefits of medical marijuana to many ailments and illnesses. The researches on the benefits of the plant are becoming increasingly interesting to many who have little means to sustain the purchase of medication. Marijuana releases dopamine in the brain helping an individual calm down, whilst causing the feelings of pleasure and relief from stress. But because of legalities and availability in some countries, marijuana is not always readily available to patients suffering from one ailment or another. Before looking to use marijuana medicinal reasons you want to make sure that it is regulated and legal to use in your area.

## Massage

For thousands of years, massage has been lauded to be a tool which detoxifies the body and a great way to just ease and relax the mind of a person. To lower your stress levels, get regular massages to calm your mind and alleviate it from urges to do ritualistic OCD actions.

## Regular Exercise

Take care of your metabolism and allow the release of healthy endorphins by means of regular exercise. It is the cheapest and easiest manner to increase these good chemicals in your body. Go, get out there and make a regimen of exercising at least 3-4 times a week. Not only does exercise do wonders for our body, it also helps distract us from the things that cause stress and anxiety. Get your blood-rate up by keeping your physical condition in tip top shape through expelling stored up energy. Doing so would likely allow you to avert OCD symptoms and behaviors. A natural stress reliever, exercise is also a good way to take care of your mental health.

## Ginko Biloba

SSRIs and other OCD medication have side effects and may affect different people in different ways. One of the side effects of OCD medication is sexual dysfunction. The herbal supplement ginko biloba can aid the patient in getting back to their lives whilst overcoming the side effects of SSRIs. Talk to your doctor about this.

## Kava Kava

Much like marijuana, kava kava is not always legaly available in some countries and are restricted in some. However the benefits of kava kava to insomnia and anxiety, some of the side effects of OCD, could help an individual suffering from the disorder to avoid compulsiveness or at the very least cut back on the severity of the disorder. Consulting with your specialist before seeking out and using kava kava will be a good discussion to have with your health care specialist.

## Gotu Kola

This very strong herbal supplement is a means for treating depression as well as anxiety. It has been used in Chinese traditional medicine as well as Ayuverdic traditions for thousands and thousands of years. Gotu kola is an ideal herbal supplement which helps individuals overcome their anxiety and OCD trigger symptoms, allowing patients to operate calmly sans the nervous tics and frequent distractions.

## St. John's Wort

St John's Wort is one of the better preferred treatments of the herbal sort that has displayed positive results on patients suffering from OCD. Taking a daily dose of the herbal medicine allows for an easy manner of reducing stress levels, allowing clarity of mind and improved mental focus. This can result in a reduction in compulsions, negative thoughts and ritualistic behavior. You do not have to go at OCD on your own. It is important there is someone you can talk to about the disorder because it studies has shown that there is a link between OCD, depression and a high probability of risk of suicide. Seek out the help of a therapist, a friend, a family member or a physician if you think you or a family member may be suffering from OCD.

## Get Sleep

Being sleep deprived can cause people to become anxious and this rate exponentially rises when a person suffering from OCD is deprived of a good night's sleep. The lack of sleep can mess with a person's clarity and sense of wellness. Set a definite time for sleeping and make sure that you stick to it. Making sure that your sleep space is conducive to good sleeping habits is a must. No computers, mobile phones or devices should flank your bed. Switch off the lights and allow yourself to relax in a comfortable bed.

Make a sleep schedule and stick to it. It may be challenging at first to follow this waking, sleeping pattern but sticking to it will allow for a better habit of sleeping and waking on time. These things will allow you to become more energized and noticeably less fatigues. Undefined and uncertain sleep patterns can equate to clinical depression making the symptoms of OCD worse.

## Quit Smoking

Smoking cigarettes are detrimental to people who siuffer from OCD, the rush and depletion as well as the addictive nature of cigarette smoking makes for a dangerous combination for those already suffering from OCS. To increase the level of patterned behavior is not a helpful thing when suffering from OCD.

# Chapter Five: Self – Help Treatment Methods

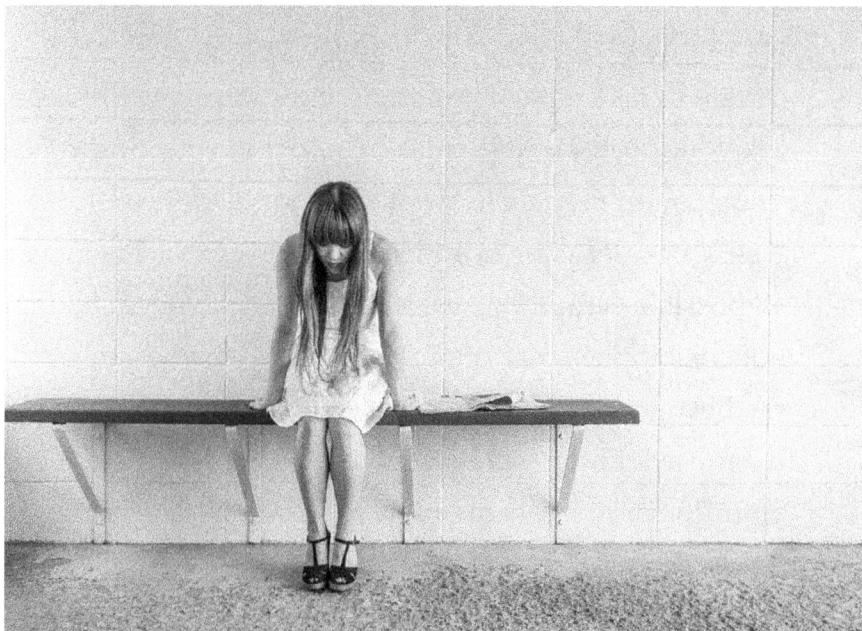

There are a number of ways an OCD patient can help themselves. One very useful and effective way to eliminate compulsive behavior is to face your fears! Avoiding your fears may lessen trigger situations but it does not help you in eliminating the behavior and could in fact worsen the scenario if you do not face it head on. In this chapter, we'll give you some tips on what you can do to help yourself and respond better to treatment. OCD can be prevented if you know how to control it. If there's a will, there's a way!

## Treatment Goals and Therapeutic Tips

Before meeting up with your specialist and as your appointment date with the medical professional nears, make certain to take note of important questions you will need to ask your doctor so as to make the best of your time together. You want to prepare answers for your doctor as well. Consider your treatment goals and jot a list of any and all possible symptoms you have displayed. Begin taking note of supplements, vitamins, herbal remedies, other medication, as well as medical conditions you have been diagnosed. These will be very important information for your doctor to know in order to find the best treatment path for you.

Your doctor will have a set of his own questions to ask you as well to help determine. Are you plagued by thoughts you cannot help but imagining? Are you compelled to keep things in a certain order. Have you noticed these episodes to be a continuing occurrence or do they happen occasional. You will be asked about symptoms you have been displaying, any experiences that may have been significant since the onset of the symptoms.

When do you remember the symptoms begin displaying? Are there occasions when the symptoms seem to worsen? Are there occasions when the symptoms seem to ease up? How do these affect your daily routine? It will be very important for your doctor to know how much time you spending a day on compulsive behavior and obsessive thoughts. Since mental is believed to have hereditary and environmental roots you will be asked about any family members who suffer from mental illness as well.

You may want to discuss the methods of how they treat OCD, the length of treatment, medication that may help if absolutely necessary. You want to find out how therapy could help your condition. Ask about methods they apply in treating OCD. You may want to ask about CBT as well as Exposure and Response Prevention therapy. Ask about what you can do in order to help yourself.

## Self – Help Therapeutic Tips

### Face Your Fears

The more a person avoids their fears the scarier it will feel for them in the long run. This may lead to a worsening of an OCD case. Challenge yourself when you are feeling brave to rise up and try to face your fears. Put yourself in a situation which exposes you to the fear of whatever it is which triggers you and then delay the desire to carry out your go-to compulsive ritual when it becomes too hard to resist the urge to complete your ritual, keep an estimate of the time you used to spend on the ritual. See your anxiety level reduce as you realize the power you have over controlling the symptoms of OCD.

## Know and Anticipate the OCD Urges

You can help yourself by knowing when to anticipate these compulsive urges before they happen. One way of doing this is by making a mental picture of what you had already completed doing. That means being in the moment of the action as you do it. Doing so allows you not to forget that the task has been completed and accomplished and will give you a sense of relief.

If you are the kind who runs around the house ten times, checking that each and every appliance is switched off, be kind to yourself and stay in the moment. Try practicing taking mental pictures of yourself as you go about these necessary chores before leaving the house.

## Redirect Your Attention

Another effective method of helping yourself when you notice a day that would more likely be a day of triggers is redirecting and refocusing your attention to something other than your thoughts. Picking up exercise is a good way not only to detoxify, get healthy but also to distract yourself from your thoughts, urges and ritualistic performances.

Distract yourself with music or a short TV series online. The aim is to distract yourself from your urges and thoughts for at least 15 minutes so that this delays the obsessive compulsion response.

## Schedule Your Worries

Learn to develop the habit of rescheduling your worries for later instead of attempting to suppress them when they arise. Devote a specific place in your home or workplace, and at least 10 minutes of your time in a day and use that time to worry about everything you worry about. Make sure that you pencil this schedule in your OCD Journal. During this time specific only to dealing with your worries, focus solely on the thought without attempting to correct it. When the period of scheduled worrying is up, make sure to breathe calming breaths and imagine the negative thought escape you as you exhale. Imagine the intrusive thoughts like a picture in watercolor and allow it to wash out of your head. Return and focus on the task at hand. Should an intrusive thought creep into your head after this, write your thoughts down instead and make a note to schedule the worry for later and go about the rest of your day.

## Keep a Journal of the Obsessive Thoughts

A person's brain suffering from OCD is like a broken record that skips and is stuck at a certain thought. Another strategy you can employ is to journal and writes about your obsessive thoughts. You want to focus on keeping a recorded document of what it is that triggered you, for one, but more importantly you want to take exact note what is running through your head at the moment as well as any phrases you might be repeating out loud or in your head, as well as any ritualistic actions or repetitive ticks and urges that follow.

You will also want to take note of how long you had tried to resist the urge and how long you spent on the ritual when you carried it out. One idea about the effectively of writing down your fears is that if you write it often enough it gets to a point where it loses its power to gain control of your thoughts. It is also much harder to concentrate on writing down thoughts than it is if you just allow them to build a picture in your head. This way the likelihood of your obsession waning sooner is higher than if you allowed it free reign on your mind.

At the end of the day, take time to reflect upon what you had written down on your worry journal. Allow yourself 10 minutes midday and 10 minutes at night to ponder over and think about them. Write down any new reactions or triggers that may occur.

## Make a Voice Recording Account of Your OCD Obsessions

Take a tape recorder, a voice recorder or a voice recorder app and document your worries, urges and fears on the device. Play the recording back and listen to it again and again for a period of about 45 minutes every day until you notice the obsession no longer grabs hold of you. You will slowly begin to notice that the fear itself has less power over you as you become less anxious. You want to repeat this exercise for every different obsession you may have.

## Educate Yourself

Educate yourself about OCD. This is not only aimed toward people who suffer from OCD, but it is also very important for family members to understand what OCD is, what role it plays in the life of a patient as well as the impact it can have on the OCD individual and their families.

There have been many instances in the past where families and family member would get to frustrated and stressed out by the disorder and has had OCD disrupt their lives. Knowing is the first thing anyone with OCD needs to do. Get informed about the disorder in order to be able to help yourself find ways to manage and control the disorder without it taking the reins of your life first.

Become an expert and get to know what you are dealing with OCD. It is a disorder which comes and goes and can happen a number of times, anytime, during your lifetime. Knowing how to deal with OCD is a requirement you should take upon yourself and your loved ones in order to be able to deal and handle situations should they come up. Make it a point to read all you can about OCD.

Search for free seminars and jump at each chance you can get to sit in and listen to one. Learning about this, often times, disabling behavioral disorder will allow you to keep the illness at bay. Discuss this with your doctor and therapist and find out all that you can about the disorder. You may also want to think about joining the Obsessive-Compulsive Foundation where a list of informative resources and recommended literature is given. Your safest and surest way to successfully managing OCD is being well informed about the illness.

You will be talking to your doctor at least once a week at the beginning of your treatment. During this time, you and your clinician will be working together closely to develop a cognitive behavioral therapy treatment plan. Aside from this, you both shall be monitoring OCD symptoms, recording, documenting and journaling will fall mostly on your shoulders as you will be the one experiencing the effects of the medication doses as well as their side effects.

Visits with your clinician, therapist or doctor will lessen once you get better. However you will still need to see your physician at least once a year. You will need to get in touch with your doctor should anything change. This is especially for severe OCD cases where therapy, medication or both have worked and later the patient experiences recurrence of the disorder.

## Quitting Treatment

Keep in mind that it is a lot more difficult to keep OCD under control than it is to have it. Since OCD is usually a lifelong illness for many, it would not be wise for you to think that there will never be a time of recurrence. And this is one reason why it is very important for people, especially those with as well as family member, living with OCD. Quitting medications or treatment without first discussing it with your doctor lest the patient runs into a relapse, the risk of relapse is always a possibility once diagnosed with OCD.

Do not be embarrassed about seeking a second opinion from another doctor about the wisdom of cognitive behavioral therapy. Consulting with a specialist about psychotherapy, medication in proper doses could greatly help the disorder. It is sometimes difficult for patients to be forthcoming with their doctors for one reason or another, so it is vital that you are aware of how important it is your doctor becomes privy information in relation to your health. Be upfront and discuss your doubts about medication or the treatments given.

It is natural for OCD patients to have doubts about their treatment once in a while. It is important that you discuss this with your therapist, doctor or family member. Do not get too surprised if you begin to find treatments disconcerting or if side effects start displaying a couple of weeks after you begin taking them. This is when journaling about your medication and doses as well as its effects on you on a daily basis.

Should you feel that the prescribed drug given to you is not doing its job, do not attempt to change the dosage levels nor should you change the stop taking the medication. It goes the same should you begin feeling unpleasant side effects of the drug. As previously mentioned here, it could take more than a couple of tries before both you and your therapist find the best drug to treat and manage the OCD. You and your doctor will be able to work together in order to find the medication that works the best for you.

# Chapter Six: How Family and Friends Can Help

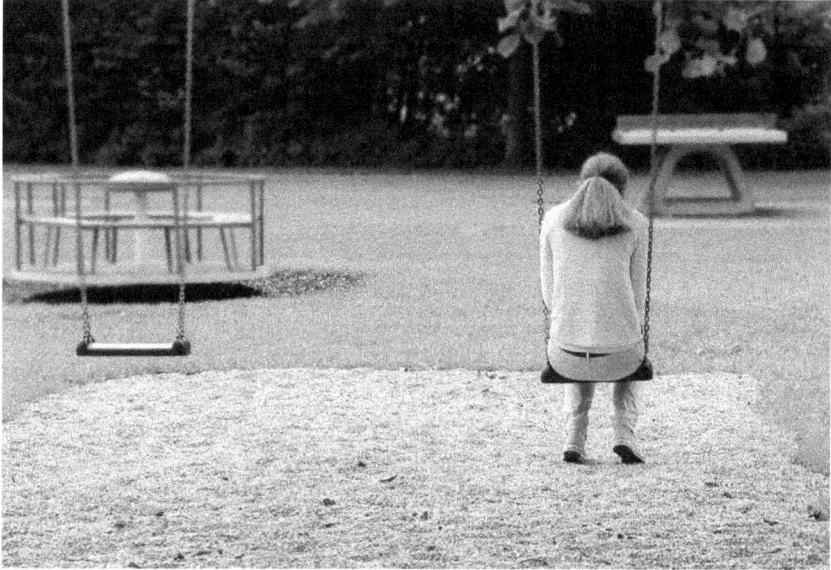

Living with OCD can be taxing too many, and it can disrupt people's lives in a big way that the family dynamics change. Many feel confused and frustrated with OCD symptoms. Should you be one of those people in the position of living with someone with OCD, your first line of defense if learning about OCD and what sort of affects it has on the patient as well as the implications it has for other family members. In this chapter, we'll give you some tips on how you can help them and support them so that they can recover and have a more positive treatment result.

## OCD by the Numbers

Obsessive - Compulsive Behavior is one among the 20 causes of disability worldwide, the World Health Organization stated in a 2001 mental health report. It was reported that OCD is the fourth most typically diagnosed mental illness trailing major depression, phobias, drug and alcohol abuse.

It is thought that OCD has a neurobiological basis. An imbalance or an abnormality, in neurotransmitters, is thought to be the culprit in OCD. Neuroimaging research show that the brain works differently in people with the disorder. It is more common for boys to have OCD during childhood than girls. Girls usually get it later in their lives. There is a close tie between adult male and females with OCD. OCD could be caused by neurological, environmental, cognitive, behavioral, and genetic factors.

OCD is considered a familial disorder if it runs in the family. Those with relations of recent who suffer from OCD are likelier themselves to develop OCD. No gene has been singled out as the culprit of OCD but with a 27-47 % of contributory genetic factors determines the truth suggesting that OC symptoms are likely to be inheritable.

OCD Symptoms in children which happen overnight may be a rooted in a Group A streptococcal infections. Group A streptococcal infections cause dysfunction and inflammation in the basal ganglia. These are referred to as pediatric autoimmune neuropsychiatric disorders; more recently though it has been identified that the bacteria with causes Lyme disease as well as the flu virus H1N1 are also closely associated to the overnight occurrence of OCD in youngsters.

Technology and brain imaging methods have given researchers the edge in detecting abnormal activity in the brain of those suffering from OCD. It has allowed the twin observation of a non-OCD patient's brain alongside the scan of one who has OCD. It is believed that an imbalance of glutamate and or serotonin could be partially responsible for OCD.

When a person has the tendency, as in genetic, to developing the condition environmental factors that weigh down as stress may be the trigger for OCD later in life. Studies has found that around 30 percent of young children ages 6-18 and has experienced some sort of traumatic brain injury could develop OCD symptoms. Studies reveal that

OCD symptoms later in a person's life are reported to have started after a traumatic brain injury. Refusing to go to school is a widespread mental health issue concerning a lot of people. Up to 5% of youth display school refusal traits which concern and affect their parents, caregivers and guardians. Teachers included.

School absenteeism is linked to a spike in numbers of developmental disorders and psychiatric problems in adulthood.There have been good results which propose that a comprehensive treatment approach, like behavioral parent management training, cognitive-behavioral treatment of an individual, and working with school staff can help move on and promote a more stable and normal school attendance record for young people who refuse to attend school due to anxiety.

Here is an overview of cognitive-behavioral treatment in relation to school refusal and school-related anxiety.

- You first need to identify the functions of school refusal. Find out and investigate what is making the child refuse to go to school. Was there an embarrassing incident that happened lately? Where there any changes in the class roster like a new teacher who joined the ranks or a new classmate who may have impacted the child's unawares in the recent past?

- Assess a cognitive-behavioral approach for the child who exhibits school refusal behavior by talking to your healthcare specialist about this. Find out if there is reason to believe that the symptoms being displayed by the child is due to OCD.

- Provide parents with plans aiming at getting better and more successful results in in effectively having the child's return back to school. Cooperate and Work closely with school staff and other mental health providers to coordinate a care plan.

## How You Can Help Patients with OCD

Not only should you learn more about OCD, the person with OCD should be able to know more about the behavioral disorder as well. There are many educational materials out there about OCD that give extensive, in - depth information about the illness. Look for informative reading materials which give practical tips aimed to help family members of those living with OCD learn to cope.

Some people with OCD are and may be reluctant to talk about it with family or friends for fear of being labeled crazy. OCD does not mean that a person is mad. The lack of serotonin to a person's brain is what causes OCD and there are many factors like genetics, environment and possibly other illnesses with cause OCD. The first step to getting better is to understand that there are available treatments and no they are not mad.

A person who is clearly showing symptoms of OCD but is in denial of the fact is a lot harder to convince to see a doctor or seek treatment. Continue to leave around educational material about OCD so as the person with the illness has easy access to them. Leave them out in the open so that anyone can, most especially the one with OCD can read it when no one is around and looking over their shoulder. It could be helpful to have the family sit down for a meeting to talk about the problem similar to how one would approach someone if they were facing an alcohol problem and is in denial.

The manner of how individual family members react to the symptoms can greatly affect the disorder. If all the members of the family were in on the same page this would not be an issue at all. But for others it is not quite the same. OCD can cause a great deal of family disruptions, frustration and other problems for the family because of the rituals they are tied up to when one member of the family is suffering from OCD. In some cases family members will be advised to go in for therapy and counseling as well. Keep in mind though those family problems aren't the causes of OCD but how each family member reacts to the symptoms.

A calm support group is essential to the wellbeing and the positive results of treatment for a person with OCD. The support of a loving family can fast track the improved outcome of a treatment for an individual with OCD, whilst criticism, negative comments and snarky remarks could just worsen the situation as well as the symptoms. The best way to help is to approach the OCD behavior and patient with kindness. Simply telling a person with OCD to stop doing what they do when the compulsive behavior could make the person just feel worse because they are not able to follow.

Focus instead on the strengths of the person and praise all successful attempts of the person who resist their OCD responses. Make sure that you not expect too much that you push a person too hard, or too little that you allow the person to relapse. A good thing to keep in mind is that no one hates OCD more than the person who has it themselves.

If the ritualistic actions were allowed by the family to go on for some time as a manner of coping with the disorder then all the more so should they seek help as a family to unlearn the things they have allowed themselves to become accustomed. A therapist will be able to guide each family member to disentangle themselves from being participants in the rituals, with the knowledge and consent of the patient. Should you "cold-turkey" an OCD individual from your participation in what was once usual to them, this may cause more imbalance to the OCD patient and set the family two steps back from recovery.

It is never good to just drop a surprise like that on a person whose illness is finding their balance through the rituals they carry out since they will not be able to manage the distress. When you abruptly refuse to participate with the rituals of the patient with their consent, it will only set the patient back more. It will certainly not help the patient discover a long - term strategy to cope with the OCD symptoms and they may just withdraw into themselves. Do not ignore this fact.

It is important to work as a team and have everyone in the family well aware of the condition of living with OCD behavior. Be aware of telltale signs of a relapse because you may notice this before the person with OCD does. If the symptoms of the illness does start displaying for a person who has recovered sit down point out the symptoms in a caring manner and drop a suggestion of discussing it with a doctor. Family members will have to learn to tell the difference between a bad day and OCD.

If a family member is undergoing treatment for OCD it is also important for other concerned family members to talk to the doctor about the treatment. This is because family members are usually present in the day of the life of the person in treatment and can be another source of information on how the patient is responding to medication. Family members are also the first ones to notice how the patient tries to help themselves by delaying responses and confirm it with the clinician. Be encouraging with the patient and remind them to be religious about taking their medication and support during CBT treatments.

On the other hand, be mindful about improvements. If an OCD patient has been undergoing treatment for a fair amount of time without positive results or perhaps there are worrying side effects stemming from medications, accompany them to the doctor and say so. You may want to look at other medication and therapy available or you can get a second opinion too.

Working with schools and teachers will be very important for parents who have a child with OCD because they too will need to understand what OCD is. Parents will have to set consistent boundaries, letting the child or juvenile know what is expected from them.

There are many support groups and help out there where family members of people with OCD can get help. Sometimes, just talking with a group can be a big help in taking off some of the frustration that comes along with OCD. Support groups are meant to make a person feel less alone as they learn new ways to cope and assist the family member with OCD.

If you are a family member, or living with a friend with OCD, make sure that you have time for yourself. Take turns checking in on a family member who may have severe OCD so that no one person is laden with the task on their own. You will be a better support link for your loved one if you take care of yourself too.

# Chapter Seven: Other Treatment Options

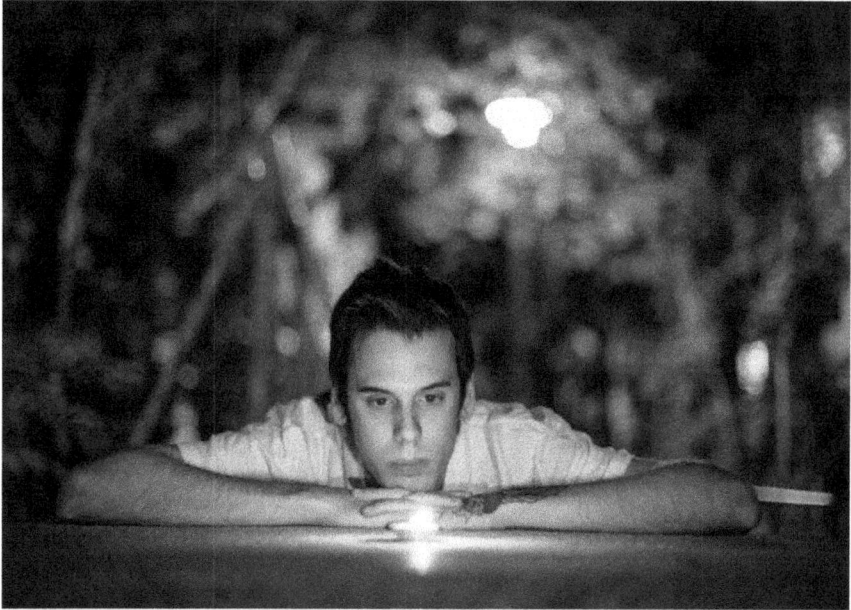

Cognitive behavioral psychotherapy is the preferred OCD treatment for children, juveniles and adults alike. There is a consistent relationship amongst the targeted outcome, the treatment and the disorder which aids the patient in internalizing as they focus on a strategy to resist OCD. Behavior therapy helps OCD patients to change their feelings and thoughts by changing their behavior first. Exposure and response prevention is a behavior therapy method used in treating OCD.

## Cognitive Behavioral Psychotherapy

When a person is faced with their fears often enough in small doses on a regular basis it almost usually lessens the anxiety in the person. Coming into contact with something feared in small controlled doses allows the individual with OCD to be exposed in a safe space until their anxiety diminishes. One example is the fear of contamination by germs and virus. A person with OCD could be asked to handle money or be exposed to objects handled by others, like doorknobs, until such time the patient no longer feels fear of contact.

In order for this therapy to be optimal in treatment it has to be combined with ritual prevention where the person with OCD blocks the avoidance behavior and rituals or at least delays it until such time that the ritualistic behaviors are completely out the person. Exposure addresses the issue of obsessions and anxiety whilst ritual prevention helps decrease the instances of compulsive behaviors. Many people who suffer from OCD have reportedly had little difficulty in tolerating the combination of Cognitive Behavioral Therapy and Ritual Prevention once they have begun.

Different people react to psychotherapy differently just as they would to medication. Most OCD patients get anxious during treatment however, cognitive behavioral therapy is relatively free of side effects unlike medicating alone. CBT sessions can be requested to be done on a one on one basis or individual CBT where the patient works with the doctor alone. Another sort of CBT session is group CBT, where the sessions are done with doctor, patient and family or friends.

Doctors may give both medications side by side with cognitive behavioral therapy. On the other hand, a social worker or a psychologist may carry out the CBT sessions whilst a doctor manages the administration, prescription and monitoring medications. Whatever the specialties of the individual health provider, the people giving an OCD patient has to be knowledgeable in relation to the treatments given to the patient. They should be willing to work closely with you in providing mental care.

## Cognitive Therapy

Another component of cognitive behavioral therapy is CT or cognitive therapy. Cognitive therapy usually goes along with exposure and ritual prevention therapy in order to lessen the catastrophic manner of thinking and burden of responsibility frequently displayed by people with OCD. Let's cite an example; say, a young child may believe that her failure to remind her father to wear a seatbelt could, in the mind of the child, ultimately get the father in an accident and die on that day. Cognitive therapy can help the child understand and challenge the wrong ideas in their obsessive thought to help improve their way of responding to the obsessive thought.

Some of the other techniques used in psychotherapy are a method called distraction and stopping the OCD symptom; a method wherein the patient suppresses or switches off the symptoms and response to the disorder. Another is called "satiation" wherein the patient listens to a closed-loop audio recording of their obsession until the thought loses its power grip on the individual. Habit reversal is when a patient is asked to replace a ritualistic behavior with a closely similar but non-OCD behavior, paying mind to create new habits outside of the disorder. And lastly, a helpful but not as efficient method than the standard CBT is contingency management; this method uses rewards as an incentive to ritualistic behaviors.

You will want to get the most out of your psychotherapy sessions by first showing up for your appointment sessions. Another thing you want to remember is to be upfront, open and honest with your doctor and or social worker. To get the most out of your sessions and to help yourself along during treatment, patients are encouraged to do their homework and learn about OCD that is part of your therapy treatment. Do not forget to give your doctor, social worker or therapist feedback about how your treatment is going, whether you think it is working or not, taking note to mention any disturbing or uncomfortable side effects of the medication given to you.

The success rate of CBT is promising for those who complete the therapy. Those who accomplish 12-20 session say there is a 50 to 80% noticeable reduction in OCD symptoms. Importantly, those suffering from OCD and respond to CBT well stay well for years to come. CBT alongside taking medication could help the prevention of a relapse once prescription medication is stopped.

It may take up to about 2 months or more for CBT, when carried out on a weekly basis, to display its full effects. The quickest treatment for OCD takes around 2-3 hours of therapist or doctor assisted exposure, ritual prevention sessions for a period of 3 weeks.

When rare cases of severe OCD are presented to doctors or therapists, the CBT sessions are usually carried out in a hospital setting. Many patients do well with intermittent, gradual CBT on a weekly basis. They in turn are told to go about the rest of the week with homework to do. Homework usually involves exposing oneself to objects or situations which trigger the OCD symptoms. Since these triggers and symptoms are unique to each patient, it is often challenging to reproduce these scenarios in a doctor's office. There are instances when a therapist could pay a visit to the patient in the workplace or at home to carry out exposure, ritual prevention sessions.

## How to Find a CBT Psychotherapist

Finding a trained cognitive-behavioral psychotherapist may prove to be difficult depending on the location of your residence. It is especially challenging to find a seasoned one who has shown success in working with juveniles and children. In order to locate a therapist who is skilled and learned in the administration of CBT for OCD patients, the first person you want to discuss it with and approach is your family physician, which may be able to give you recommendations of skilled CBT therapists. You can also go to a school and ask the psychiatry or psychology department of the local academic school. There are many local support groups that are scattered everywhere in the country, you may want to look into that and ask around your area of residence where you can find a therapist. Ask around and locate your local OCD support group. There are also other ways of finding a good therapist if you check out The Anxiety Disorders of America, the Obsessive Compulsive Foundation, or the Association for the Advancement of Behavioral Therapy.

There are cases where you would be able to locate local cognitive behavioral psycho therapists in your area who have experience with depression and or anxiety but may have little no to no experience with OCD. With the many reading materials and literature available on OCD, you may want to find a therapist wiling to learn the methods of CBT. This is for when there is no readily available therapist with the experience working with OCD patients needing CBT treatments. Find one who is willing to learn the skills and methods of CBT since it is quite simple to translate CBT methods and skills from one disorder to CBT.

## Other Important Reminders

Keep in mind that CBT involves exposure and ritual prevention by way of working on a list of your OCD symptoms, ranked from easiest to most difficult to resist. If you feel you are not being administered the proper sort of CBT treatment sessions, do not be embarrassed to seek a second opinion. If this is the case, then ultimately, driving out to a center which specializes in intensive CBT sessions, whether on an inpatient or outpatient basis, could be the solution that is best for you to look into and more practical in the long run. You want to be able to use the time you have at sessions toward progressive treatment and not waste time, energy or money.

Effective medication for OCD is presently available in the market. These medications raise the serotonin concentration levels. Serotonin is a chemical responsible for communicating with the brain. Right now there are five serotonin reuptake inhibitors, also called SRI, which work well in treating OCD namely; Clomipramine, Fluoxetine,

Fluvoxamine, Paroxetine, and Sertraline. Of the five available prescription OCD medications, the only nonselective SRI is Clomipramine. This equates to the medication affecting a lot of other neurotransmitter aside from serotonin and it has more complicated side effects than the four other medications mentioned above which solely SSRIs are. This is why most therapist and doctors prescribe SSRIs first because these drugs are usually easier to tolerate than the nonselective SRI drug.

A moderate improvement, after a period of 8-10 weeks, will most usually be reported by patients in therapy and undergoing medication using SRI drugs. Those being treated with medication alone have a lesser chance of not getting OCD symptoms than those who underwent therapy and medication combined together. This is the reason why medication and therapy, when done correctly, is strongly advised by physicians and therapists, because of the lasting results of the combined treatment using both therapy and medication. There is also a likelihood that around 20% of OCD patients will not respond to a particular SRI. If this is the case, tell your doctor and ask them of the other SSRI medications still available to you.

Research has shown that all the SRI drugs are equally effective. Side effects however are lesser when a patient's treatment is started off with one of those medications.

This information will be good to know, most especially if a previous family member has had the experience of not responding well to a particular medication in the past. Drugs interacting with other drugs are a possibility. This is why it is important for your doctor to know of other conditions an OCD patient has such as sleeping or stomach problems or if the patient is taking other medications for other medical conditions. Your doctor would be better able to recommend other SSRIs to reduce the possibility of the drugs interacting with one another.

The possibility that the first drug prescribed to a patient will not take effect immediately. Patient reports state that individuals would usually feel and notice some of the drug's benefits after about 3 to 4 weeks. Optimum benefits to taking the medication usually and should happen after about 10 to 12 weeks by means of adequate medication dosage. If after this period of time the patient reports and displays no response to the medication, seasoned physicians would most usually prescribe any of the SRIs.

As much as SRIs work equally well, there is also a factor to the make-up of each individual and how they respond to medication. SRIs, as with clomipramine, are generally more tolerated by most individuals, despite the minor side effects like dizziness, weight gain, sedation, and dry mouth that come along with it. On the other hand, the other 4 SSRIs (sertraline, fluvoxamine, fluoxetine and paroxetine) possess the same side effects which include nausea, diarrhea, nervousness, restlessness and insomnia. All five drugs are known to likely cause sexual dysfunction problems but more often than not cases are higher when the patient in question has been taking clomipramine.

Children, juveniles and adults who suffer from OCD with a preexisting heart condition or disease will need to undergo an electrocardiogram test before taking clomipramine because this drug has a high likelihood of causing blood pressure problems as well as irregular heartbeats. ECGs should be tested at intervals for the duration of the patients' treatment to analyze if there is cause for concern.

Side effects stem from the dose of medication taken and the length of time a patient has been taking it. It is vital that doctors and patients work hand in hand and start low doses of medication, increasing the dose slowly thereafter. Severe side effects of these drugs are usually attributed to large doses and/or a sudden increase of dosage. In the long run patients develop better tolerance for the side effects stemming from the SSRIs than they would with clomipramine. Save from fluoxetine all SRIs has to be tapered and ceased gradually due to the probability of symptoms returning as to avoid reactions of withdrawal to the drug. Be mindful of your reactions to the drug and write these, if any, in your OCD symptoms and treatment journal. Be sure that this is discussed with your therapist or doctor.

Because we are all individuals with different make ups, people have varied side effects from medication. Some side effects from medication, like sleepiness, could aid one person and be disruptful for another. The side effects one could get would depend on the amount and kind of medication you take, your age, existing medical conditions you may have, your body chemistry and other medication you may be taking. Again it is important for your doctor to ask about your medical background and equally important for you to be upfront honest and proactively contributing to detecting other illnesses for which you may be taking other medication.

Should side effects become an issue or intrude on your schedule and daily life your doctor can try a number of things to help you out. Your doctor may try reducing the intake of medication. By gradually decreasing the dose the aim is to get to a dose low enough that it reduces the ill effects of the side effect, but not too low that it causes a relapse. Should the side effects be intruding on your sleep (insomnia) or sexual problems, your doctor may add another medication to help the side effects along. Your doctor could also try a different medicine to figure out if there are lesser if not more tolerable side effects. Even if a drug is clearly doing its job but entails side effects that are intolerable for an individual, trying out another drug is a sound plan.

This is not something a patient wants to carry out on their own, changing medications on our own without the advice of your doctor can be very risky. Never attempt to lower or increase your medication dose on your own. Do not change the medication without discussing it with your doctor and most especially do not go ahead in switching up your medication for another if the doctor has already advised against it. You will have to discuss any problems related to the medication given by your doctor with them.

Should little benefit be reflected after a 6 week period of medication, you might want to discuss adding cognitive behavioral therapy to your treatment. Sometimes another medication along with the SRI can be helpful too. Most medical experts are on the same page about CBT being the most helpful treatment when a patient with OCD does not respond to medication on its own, avoidance of situations that set off anxiety or continuing with OCD rituals only blocks off the effects of the medication. In order for medication to take effect and to see actual results, a patient diagnosed with OCD has to imperatively attempt to resist their ritualistic tendencies. The addition of CBT on top of the medication given to and taken by the patient aids treatment along because it teaches the OCD patient to expose themselves to things and situations which trigger the OCD symptoms which they have to resist performing.

For those who have higher anxiety levels than others adding a medication to reduce anxiety to the SRI could help. Anti-anxiety drugs include sorts like alprazolam or clonazepam.

When thought-disorder or tics are the problematic areas of a patient, drugs containing a high potency neuroleptic like risperidone or haloperidol could be useful in treatment. These medications are more complex in its mix therefore is reserved for individuals who have not shown much of an improvement with medications alongside CBT.

Your doctor will need enough time to come to any conclusions about the efficacy or the non-responsiveness of an OCD patient to a treatment very little consensus on what to do next when a patient with OCD does not respond to properly carried out CBT alongside a proper administration of sequential SRI trials. Switching clomipramine from an SSRI could help improve the treatment of a previously non responsive patient. Experts would usually prescribe a clomipramine trial after 2 or 3 SSRI trial failures. There are instances when a combination of an SSRI and clomipramine is used either to help elevate the benefits of a medication or reduce its side effects.

An adult experiencing unremitting and extremely severe OCD, interrupting specified malfunctioning brain circuits, through neurosurgical treatment can be helpful. Other patients with severe OCD alongside with depression can benefit from electroconvulsive therapy (ECT).

Medical specialists treating pregnant women or women planning on becoming pregnant prefer to opt for cognitive behavioral therapy alone as treatment. However, because OCD typically worsens during the period of pregnancy, medication may be necessary. It is however advised that the woman use medication sparingly and under the supervision of their doctor. Clomipramine is not a choice doctors would give to a woman who has intentions of getting pregnant and more so for women who are expecting experts who deem that the pregnant or soon to be pregnant patient prescribes SSRIs instead.

SSRIs are also preferred for patients who have a preexisting or a coexisting heart disease but still need medication. The same is to be said for OCD patients with renal failure.

Should a patient display another psychiatric disorder, your physician will most likely mix and match medication treatments for the other conditions. In some cases, the same medication could be administered for two different disorders. An example would be an SRI for panic disorder and OCD. On the other hand, more than one medication will be needed for more complex cases like OCD and concurrent mania when an SRI and mood stabilizers are needed. Lab tests are not necessary when given any one of the SSRIs available but will be required before commencing the administration clomipramine. Although not addictive, it is always recommended to gradually cease taking SRIs.

Most people with OCD can usually be treated as outpatients. However, in some cases of severe OCD involving aggressive impulses or depression it may be necessary to hospitalize the person for their safety. A person who possesses a really severe case of OCD or if the OCD is further complicated by a neuropsychiatric or a medical condition, admission into hospital can be a good avenue to take in order to introduce intensive CBT care. Medication really depends on the gravity of the OCD a patient has. Another factor in medication administration is the age of the individual.

# Bonus Chapter:

## Famous People Who Have OCD

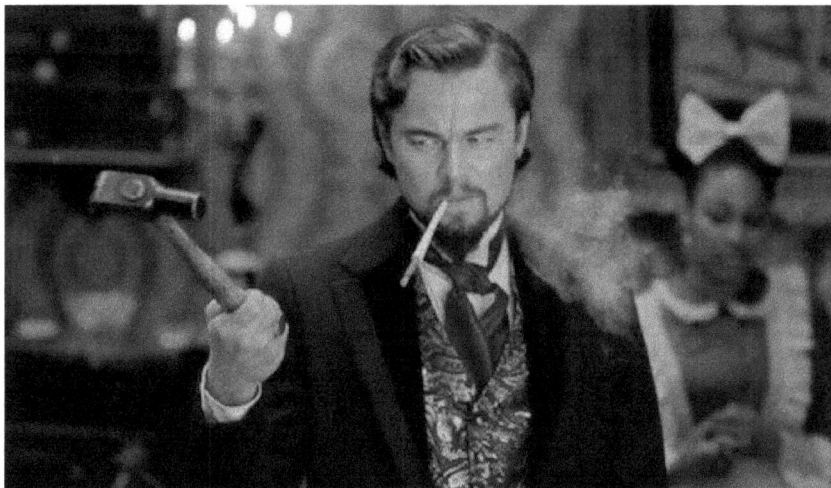

We have discussed some of the medications, available therapy as well as alternative ways that patients with OCD have available to them, this time let us look at some individuals who are familiar to us by way of the small and big screens who have been battling their way through with OCD. OCD chooses randomly and respect not the status, age, gender of a person. It can be an incredible burden for those who suffer from it because it takes away time, energy and focus away from what needs to be minded. However this doesn't mean that you can't do it!

## Notable Celebrities and Artists Battling OCD

Many have succeeded in warding off the symptoms of OCD and so can you. Mental illness has been at the forefront lately and has been on many headlines banners, talked about in shows and is found on many print materials. Famous people are not spared of the disorder either as you will see in the following segment.

### Megan Fox

The Jennifer's Body lead actress has reportedly been one of the celebrities who came out and openly discussed her battle with OCD. The leading lady of Transformers has come out to talk about her fight with OCD and has given light to how a patient suffering from the disorder can overcome the symptoms of the disorder.

Imagine being a patient with OCD and having to dive in mud, muck and grime and it can be quite a horrific thought for most patients, but Megan is one person who is testament that a person suffering from OCD can overcome their fears and ritualistic behaviors.

## Marc Summers

The Nickelodeon mainstay has somehow managed to survive the cascading green slime attack along with the mess. The host of the Double Dare show would immediately rush to have a shower after the show and then once again once he reached the confines of his home.

Allowing him to operate on a social level was his openness to getting help through a combination of therapy and medication.

## Cameron Diaz

Ms. Diaz is one of the more outspoken public figures in Hollywood who has talked about her disorder. her compulsion is manifested through her fear of germs most especially on door knobs. The Charlie's Angels actress insists on opening door using her elbows because of contamination fears. She meticulously cleans her home each day and is a compulsive hand washer. Cameron has managed to control her OCD refusing to allow it to take control of her life.

## Justine Timberlake

It may be interesting to imagine how Justine and Cameron, who once dated each other, went through their days suffering from the same disorder. A self-diagnosed OCD individual with attention-deficit disorder, Justine has admittedly some behaviors which qualify him as an OCD patient. The Sexy Back singer has compulsions of having everything in order and making sure that he is not for want for some of the foods he requires.

## Howie Mandell

One of the X Factor hosts and the main of the game show Deal or No Deal, Howie has been one of the more outspoken individuals about his OCD. Sometimes laughed at for what seem to be quirky antics is in fact a severe case of OCD. The much loved host and comic has suffered OCD for many years and has been able to rally on with help, not only from others but mainly from himself. Howie will not touch money, handrails or door knobs. Make-up artists are required to use new sponges each day when putting on his make-up and he will normally refuse to shake hands with people opting instead for a fist bump.

## David Beckham

It may come as a surprise to most that the once mud-kicking, dirt-carrying football star David Beckham is an OCD sufferer but keep in mind that the ritualistic behaviors and tics of OCD is different with each person. The dapper Beckham gets agitated when things are not arranged to his liking and when stuff is out of order. He has even been seen to arrange hotel furniture around to satisfy his OCD. Odd numbers are also a cause of concern and upset to the superstar. Living with OCD has not been easy for the husband of Victoria but he claims that not giving in to his compulsions is even more upsetting.

## Leonardo DiCaprio

The Titanic and The Great Gatsby star has been suffering from OCD since he was a child. His compulsions dictated that he step on every gum stain and jump over cracks on the street. As much as he has done to overcome the ritualistic tendencies of OCD the actor admits that there are instances when the disorder plagues and overwhelms him out of nowhere. He had actually tapped into his OCD whilst playing the part of Howard Hghes, another OCD patient.

## Howard Stern

The shock-jock has always been open about his fear of germs as well as his compulsion to think about catastrophic thoughts. Once out of college the X Factor host/radio host, his anxiety was manifested in a series of obsessive rituals and events which he writes about in his book Ms. Universe. One of the rituals he did then was to tap his car radio a certain number of times before turning it on and driving out of a lot.

## Billy Bob Thornton

The Bad Santa lead actor has had OCD most of his life and has continued to be one of his greatest worries. Also a sufferer of dyslexia, Billy Bob attributes his OCD to abusive childhood experiences, his OCD manifest in thought counting and repetition. He has been seen to take out and put in mail in his mailbox three times before actually retrieving them. Mentally, he allots "numbers" to people and mentally addresses them as such. He has even gone as far as writing a song about his disorder titled "Always Counting."

## Fiona Apple

OCD has been to blame for length of time it took for Fiona Apple to complete her latest album. The singer who soared to great heights in the early nineties has pretty severe OCD which has deemed her to live a life of recluse. Her obsessive-compulsive disorder manifests in ways that would cripple the life of a regular person. Apple has trouble driving and rarely gets out of the confines of her home. This in turn has caused her to live like a hermit.

**Lena Dunham**

Actress Lena Dunham of the HBO Original "Girls" has been an outspoken advocate of mental health wellness and battling OCD. The writer has struggled with the disorder for as long as she can remember and attributes her being able to manage and control the symptoms of OCD, through the supportive love of her parents. She gives credit to her parents for being forward thinkers, and for addressing the OCD by searching for therapy and medication. Of OCD, Lena says that there is not enough talk about the mental health wellness of a lot of people these days.

Despite the fact that mental disorders are talked about more now openly, the actress-writer feels there is more that can be said and done to shed light on these debilitating mental conditions.

# Index

# Photo References

Page 8 Photo by user johnhain via Pixabay.com, https://pixabay.com/en/brain-mind-thoughts-games-gaming-954817/

Page 12 Photo by user airpix via Flickr.com, https://www.flickr.com/photos/144152028@N08/35446304120/

Page 24 Photo by user Janine via Flickr.com, https://www.flickr.com/photos/pinkcotton/3897617882/

Page 32 Photo by user geralt via Pixabay.com, https://pixabay.com/en/despair-alone-being-alone-archetype-513529/

Page 54 Photo by user THX0477 via Flickr.com, https://www.flickr.com/photos/59195512@N00/3786033447/

Page 65 Photo by user Ryan McGuire via Pixabay.com, https://pixabay.com/en/worried-girl-woman-waiting-sitting-413690/

Page 76 Photo by user Antranias via Pixabay.com, https://pixabay.com/en/person-woman-girl-alone-409127/

Page 88 Photo by user brenkee via Pixabay.com, https://pixabay.com/en/candle-guy-young-man-male-adult-1281245/

Page 106 Photo by user 22860 via Flickr.com, https://www.flickr.com/photos/ofsmallthings/8373071753/

# References

Can Medical Marijuana be used to treat OCD? -
BeyondOcd.org
http://beyondocd.org/medical-marijuana-ocd-treatment/

Information for Friends and Family: When Someone You
Love Has OCD - BeyondOcd.org
http://beyondocd.org/information-for-friends-and-family

Living With: OCD (Obsessive Compulsive Disorder) -
PsychGuides.com
https://www.psychguides.com/guides/living-with-ocd-
obsessive-compulsive-disorder/

Obsessive - Compulsive Disorder - Webmd.com
https://www.webmd.com/mental-health/obsessive-
compulsive-disorder#1

OCD (Obsessive-Compulsive Disorder) - PsychGuides.com
https://www.psychguides.com/guides/ocd-obsessive-
compulsive-disorder/

Obsessive-Compulsive Disorder (OCD) - HelpGuide.org
https://www.helpguide.org/articles/anxiety/obssessive-
compulsive-disorder-ocd.htm

Obsessive-Compulsive Disorder Treatment Program Options - PsychGuides.com
https://www.psychguides.com/guides/obsessive-compulsive-disorder-treatment-program-options/

Related Conditions: Disorders That May Co-exist with OCD - BeyondOcd.org
http://beyondocd.org/ocd-facts/related-conditions

SELF HELP FOR OCD: Obsessive Compulsive Disorder – Get.gg
https://www.get.gg/ocd.htm

Treatments for OCD: Cognitive- behavioural therapy – CAMH.ca
http://www.camh.ca/en/hospital/health_information/a_z_mental_health_and_addiction_information/obsessive_compulsive_disorder/obsessive_compulsive_disorder_information_guide/Pages/ocd_treatments.aspx

What is Obsessive Compulsive Disorder? - AnxietyBC.com
https://www.anxietybc.com/parenting/obsessive-compulsive-disorder

What is Obsessive Compulsive Disorder? - Psychiatry.org
https://www.psychiatry.org/patients-families/ocd/what-is-obsessive-compulsive-disorder

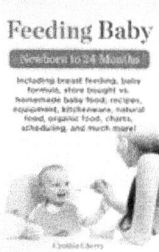

Feeding Baby
Cynthia Cherry
978-1941070000

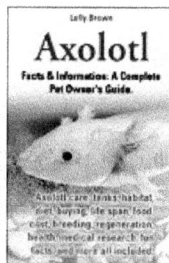

Axolotl
Lolly Brown
978-0989658430

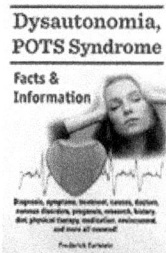

Dysautonomia, POTS
Syndrome
Frederick Earlstein
978-0989658485

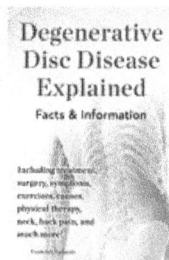

Degenerative Disc
Disease Explained
Frederick Earlstein
978-0989658485

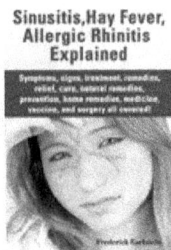

Sinusitis, Hay Fever,
Allergic Rhinitis Explained
Frederick Earlstein
978-1941070024

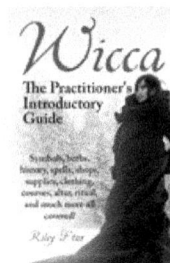

Wicca
Riley Star
978-1941070130

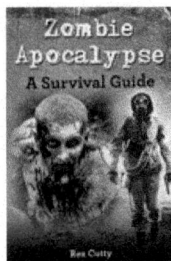

Zombie Apocalypse
Rex Cutty
978-1941070154

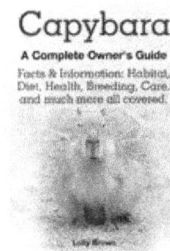

Capybara
Lolly Brown
978-1941070062

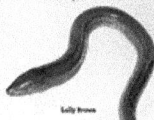

Eels As Pets
Lolly Brown
978-1941070167

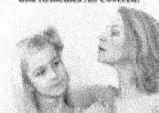

Scabies and Lice Explained
Frederick Earlstein
978-1941070017

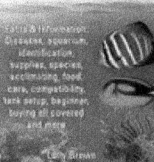

Saltwater Fish As Pets
Lolly Brown
978-0989658461

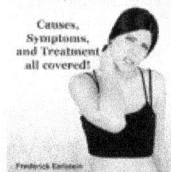

Torticollis Explained
Frederick Earlstein
978-1941070055

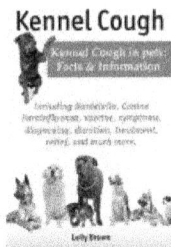

Kennel Cough
Lolly Brown
978-0989658409

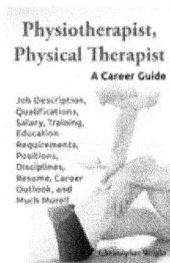

Physiotherapist, Physical
Therapist
Christopher Wright
978-0989658492

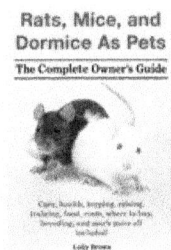

Rats, Mice, and Dormice
As Pets
Lolly Brown
978-1941070079

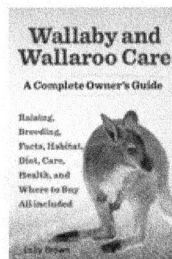

Wallaby and Wallaroo Care
Lolly Brown
978-1941070031

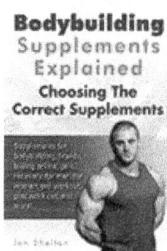

Bodybuilding Supplements
Explained
Jon Shelton
978-1941070239

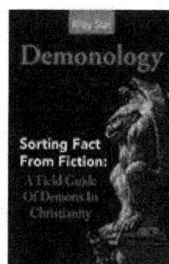

Demonology
Riley Star
978-19401070314

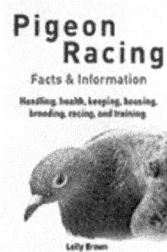

Pigeon Racing
Lolly Brown
978-1941070307

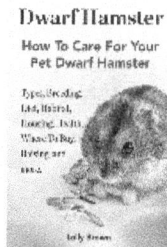

Dwarf Hamster
Lolly Brown
978-1941070390

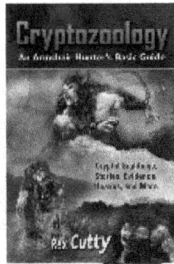

Cryptozoology
Rex Cutty
978-1941070406

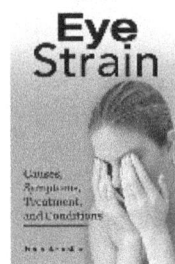

Eye Strain
Frederick Earlstein
978-1941070369

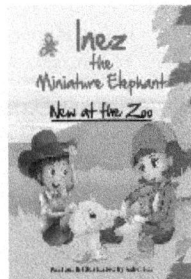

Inez The Miniature Elephant
Asher Ray
978-1941070353

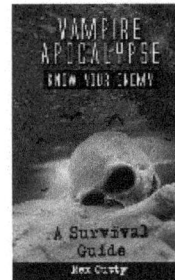

Vampire Apocalypse
Rex Cutty
978-1941070321

www.ingramcontent.com/pod-product-compliance
Lightning Source LLC
Chambersburg PA
CBHW071159200326
41519CB00018B/5291